The Unintentional Caregiver

Practical Wisdom for Your Caregiving Journey

By Joyce Shreve

Part of the Receptive Wisdom Series

The Unintentional Caregiver
Copyright © 2025 by Joyce Shreve
All rights reserved.

No part of this publication may be reproduced, distributed, or transmitted in any form or by any means, including photocopying, recording, or other electronic or mechanical methods, without the prior written permission of the author, except in the case of brief quotations embodied in critical reviews and certain other noncommercial uses permitted by copyright law.

Published by Receptive Wisdom Publishing
ISBN: 979-8-9995445-0-6

Cover and Interior Design: Joyce Shreve

For permission or inquiries, contact: www.receptivewisdom.com

This book is a work of nonfiction based on the author's personal experiences. Names and identifying details may have been changed to protect privacy.

Disclaimer
The content in this book is intended for informational and inspirational purposes only. It is not a substitute for professional medical, legal, financial, or mental health advice. Always seek the guidance of qualified professionals regarding specific questions or concerns related to health, caregiving, legal matters, or financial planning. The author and publisher disclaim any liability, loss, or risk incurred directly or indirectly from the use or application of any information contained in this book.

Printed in the United States of America

Dedications

To my mother,

You taught me how to laugh through pain, and how to keep going even when life gets hard. Your quiet resilience still guides me, even though you're no longer physically here. This book is a tribute to everything you passed on to me.

To my daughter,

You are the reasons I learned to fight, to ask hard questions, and to never give up. Your journey has shaped mine through advocacy. I'm in awe of your strength and resilience. I am and always will be proud to be your mother.

To my grandson,

You opened a whole new chapter of love and learning in my life. Your presence has changed me in ways I never expected, and I am deeply thankful for it. Everything I do now is rooted in giving you the best possible future. You keep me moving forward.

To my husband,

You are my caregiver, my rock, and my safe space. While I've spent years caring and advocating for our family members who needed me, you quietly and faithfully held down our home life and preserved as much peace for us as possible. You held me up when I was too tired to stand. Your strength, love, and steady presence have been the foundation beneath every step I've taken. Thank you for being the best life partner I could ask for. I will always love you.

To the ones who showed up when I was running empty,

To my sister-in-law, my in-laws, and the dear friends who carried me through the hours I didn't think I could survive, this is for you. You didn't just help; you *rescued*. Whether it was a weekend getaway that gave me room to breathe, a check-in text at just the right moment, or volunteering to help when I needed it, your love arrived like a gift of grace. You saw my exhaustion and answered with action, compassion, and unwavering presence.

You didn't ask for recognition. You simply showed up—and because of that, I found strength I didn't know I had. Thank you for being the quiet heroes of my hardest chapters.

To the Source greater than myself—

In the moments when I had no words left when the weight of caregiving threatened to crush me, you met me in silence, in prayer, and many times, through the lyrics of a song on the radio. That station (KLove) my husband introduced me to became more than background noise. It became a lifeline. Those uplifting songs arrived like whispers of hope, like breadcrumbs leading me back to faith, strength, and breath.

Thank you for being my guiding light and encouragement when everything else felt uncertain. For every moment of clarity, comfort, and courage—I know where it came from.

Table of Contents

Chapter 1 What Is an Unintentional Caregiver? 1

Chapter 2 Emotional Shock & the Invisible Shift 11

Chapter 3 How to Speak "Doctor" 17

Chapter 4 Surviving the Administrative Avalanche 25

Chapter 5 Crisis Mode 35

Chapter 6 Navigating the Systems That Are Supposed to Help 43

Chapter 7: The Pivot That Changes the Journey 53

Chapter 8 Planning for the Future 65

Chapter 9 Building a Support Network (Even If You're Alone) 73

Chapter 10 Taking Care of Yourself Without Guilt 81

Chapter 11 The Self-Care Toolbox: Habits That Actually Help 91

Chapter 12 Life After Caregiving 101

A Letter to the Next Caregiver 108

About the Author 111

Acknowledgements 112

Bonus Materials & Tools 113

Additional Resources 114

Preface

My letter to you, the caregiver.

Dear Caregiver,

I never set out to become a caregiver. There was no manual. No roadmap. Just a moment when love collided with necessity—and I stepped in.

Over the years, I've cared for three generations of my family: my mother, my daughter, and now my grandson. Each journey was different. Each one stretched me in ways I never expected. But through it all, one truth remained: I had to learn as II didn't have degrees in nursing or special education. What I had was persistence, prayer, and an overflowing binder of medical notes and school forms. I learned to advocate, to ask hard questions, to read between the lines, and to keep going—even when I was exhausted or afraid.

Maybe that's where you are now. Pulled into caregiving by love, crisis, or sheer survival. Maybe you feel tired, invisible, or unsure whether you're doing enough. If so, this book is for you. It's not written by a professional. It's written by someone who's lived this life for thirty-six years and counting. Inside, you'll find stories from my caregiving journey along with tips to help you and hopefully, the comfort of being seen.

You don't have to do this alone. Let's walk through it together.

— Joyce Shreve
The Unintentional Caregiver

Chapter 1
What Is an Unintentional Caregiver?

Becoming a Caregiver Without a Map

Most of us don't apply for this job; instead, we inherit it.

There's no application form for this role. No job description, orientation, or paycheck. One day, you're simply a daughter, mother, or grandparent. Then, without warning, you're the one making medical decisions, handling paperwork, arranging transportation, providing daily care, and advocating for their needs. You've become a caregiver without any prior knowledge or preparation.

That was exactly how it happened to me.

I became an unintentional caregiver at just 16 years old when my mom began experiencing serious health complications. She had

The Unintentional Caregiver

diabetes and coronary artery disease, and I was the only one left at home to care for her. I didn't know what I was doing, but I knew I had to act. I was the one rushing her to the hospital when she couldn't breathe, sitting beside her hospital bed, and speaking to the doctors and nurses on her behalf. I stayed up late reading her test results, filling out insurance applications, and helping her understand her treatment options. I didn't call it *caregiving* at the time. I called it *being there for my mama*. However, in truth, I had already assumed the role of caregiver and patient advocate, and it changed me in ways I never expected.

Years later, the cycle was repeated with my daughter, Alex. At just 14 years old, she was diagnosed with Systemic lupus erythematosus (SLE) after weeks of pain, weight loss, and missed diagnoses. I remember sitting with her in the pediatric ICU as doctors scrambled to treat her DVT and pulmonary embolism. She almost died. I stayed by her side during every appointment, every chemo session, every new diagnosis. The emotional journey was intense, from the fear of losing her to the frustration of dealing with the healthcare system. I learned how to coordinate care between multiple specialists, decipher lab results, and fight for proper educational accommodations when she was too sick to attend school. I didn't have time to fall apart. I had to be her voice until she found her own.

And then came Tre, my grandson, who came to live with my husband and me at three and a half years old. At the time, he was nonverbal, aggressive, and struggling with severe developmental delays. Nine months later, a neurodiversity diagnosis helped us

The Unintentional Caregiver

understand how to support him. I was his primary caregiver, advocate, and support system. I navigated the disability application

process, coordinated therapies, and learned how to help a child with sensory sensitivities and behavioral challenges. Caring for Tre taught me a whole new set of caregiving skills—this time in the world of pediatric mental health and special education.

With my mom, Alex, and Tre, I entered caregiving without a roadmap. I learned through trial and error, persistence, grit, determination, and love, all of which contribute to a better quality of life. Love was the driving force behind my caregiving journey. That's what it means to be an unintentional caregiver: someone who steps into the gap not because we were trained to, but because we had to—driven by love and compassion.

The caregiving role can be lonely, exhausting, and feel invisible. However, it also serves a critical and incredible purpose. Unintentional caregivers are the glue that holds families together in crisis. We become researchers, appointment schedulers, medication trackers, insurance negotiators, and emotional anchors.

This chapter and this book are dedicated to recognizing that role and giving it the dignity it deserves. If you've ever sat in a waiting room, afraid of what comes next, if you've ever fought with an insurance company, filled out overwhelming paperwork, or stayed up all night researching symptoms, you're not "just" a family member.

You're a caregiver.

Sibling and Male Caregivers: The Forgotten Advocates

Caregiving doesn't always look like a mother caring for her child or a daughter tending to her aging parent.

Sometimes, it's a brother who rearranges his life to support a sister with disabilities.

A son quietly steps into his father's role when his mother can no longer do it alone.

A grandfather who suddenly finds himself raising a second generation.

A man who was never asked—but never walked away.

Male caregivers are everywhere. So are sibling caregivers. But they're often invisible in caregiving conversations.

They don't receive the same acknowledgment, social validation, or emotional permission to say, *"This is hard."*

Let me say this clearly:

If you are a sibling caregiver, your role is sacred.

If you are a male caregiver, your strength is no less valid.

You deserve to be seen, not just as a helper, but as *the caregiver.*

The Unintentional Caregiver

"Being a caregiver isn't about gender. It's about love. And some of the strongest, most silent advocates I've known wore sneakers, not scrubs, and carried the weight without applause."

To the brothers, sons, uncles, grandfathers, and siblings who have stepped up—thank you.

You may not have asked for the title, but you've carried it with quiet strength. Whether you're lifting a wheelchair into the trunk, attending IEP meetings on your lunch break, or holding steady through the silence, your caregiving matters.

You are not invisible to me. You are the backbone in families where others might not see it.

This section is for you—a tribute to your strength, your love, and your unseen sacrifice.

May you know you are not forgotten.

You are honored here.

The Rise of Grandparent Caregivers: A Love That Starts Over

There's a growing population of grandparents raising their grandchildren.

The reasons vary: illness, addiction, incarceration, mental health crises, death, or the child's needs being too great for the biological parent to manage alone. Sometimes it's a temporary arrangement. Sometimes it becomes permanent.

The Unintentional Caregiver

I am one of them.

Raising my grandson, Tre, wasn't part of the plan. But life doesn't always follow a script. He needed me. And I stepped in with zero hesitation. I didn't have all the answers, but I had love, grit, and years of caregiving experience. God had been preparing me for this role for a long time. And that was enough to begin.

Still, the truth is: raising grandchildren comes with unique challenges. The physical stamina it takes to keep up.

The financial strain of starting over. The emotional toll of watching your child struggle while trying to protect them.

It's layered with grief, guilt, grace, and an overwhelming love that refuses to quit. And yet… we rise.

In the United States, more than 2.7 million grandparents are raising grandchildren. Of those, nearly 1 in 5 have no parent present in the home.

Many are over 60. Some are living on fixed incomes. Others have delayed retirement, downsized their homes, or reentered the workforce. And yet—they do it. Every single day.

This isn't just parenting again. It's parenting with arthritic knees, thinning patience, and a lifetime of lived experience—now reshaped for a new generation.

Raising a grandchild is not a second chance at parenting; it's a unique opportunity to make a lasting impact.

The Unintentional Caregiver

It's a sacred act of rebuilding hope from the ashes.

To every grandparent reading this who has traded a quiet retirement for bedtime routines and school drop-offs—this is for you.

To those navigating trauma, court hearings, therapy sessions, and teenage attitudes with nothing but fierce love and a prayer—this is for you.

To the ones exhausted, overlooked, and under-supported—**please hear me:**

You are not alone. And you are not failing.

You are performing a miracle in real-time.

A Moment I Will Never Forget – Matching Purses

I didn't say it out loud, but the first time I rushed my mom to the ER, I was scared out of my mind. We had matching purses that day—a minor detail that made the nurse smile and say how sweet it was. I smiled, too, but inside, I was bracing for what the doctors might say.

A Moment I Will Never Forget – 9/11 in the Hospital

Mom was in the hospital when 9/11 happened. The world outside was crumbling, and the world inside me was already shaking. I remember the TV in her room, the nurses walking around with shock and dazed expressions, and me watching the towers fall while trying to stay present for my mom. I had to compartmentalize the fear—both for the world and for her—and just keep going.

A Moment I Will Never Forget – Crying in the Parking Lot

Years later, when my daughter was in the PICU, I cried my heart out in the parking lot. My husband held me while I sobbed, completely undone. One of Alex's nurses walked by. She didn't say anything then, but later, she told me, "You did the right thing, you never broke down in front of her." But what she didn't see was how much I wanted to. I wanted to curl up and stop pretending I was okay. But instead, I walked back into that room, took Alex's hand, and smiled as if everything was under control.

Caregiving is full of those moments—quiet strength that no one applauds, private grief that no one sees, and tiny details like matching purses that somehow hold you together just a little longer.

The Caregiving Mirror – Chapter 1: Seeing Yourself in the Role

What small moment made me realize that caregiving had begun—even if I didn't call it that at the time?

How has this invisible shift changed how I see myself?

What parts of me have changed—and which ones am I still holding onto?

The Unintentional Caregiver

What part of my loved one have I already started to grieve?

Am I honoring the kind of caregiver I am, even if I don't match the usual picture?

Have I been recognized for the caregiving role I've taken on, or have I been overlooked?

What would it mean to feel seen and validated in this role?

What have I lost that others may not even notice?

Who else in my circle might be carrying this quietly? Can I reach out to them?

Chapter 2
Emotional Shock & the Invisible Shift

When Your Role Changes but No One Names It

You don't decide to become a caregiver. It begins slowly—so quietly, in fact, that most of us don't realize it's happened until we're already deep in it. It starts with one appointment. Then another. A few extra responsibilities. A dozen new questions no one warned you you'd need to answer. At first, you're just being helpful. Then you're needed. Then you're essential. And then, somehow, you're "the one."

Your title hasn't changed. Your pay doesn't change. But everything else does.

Give It a Name

One of the most empowering things you can do is name your role. When no one else says the words out loud, it can leave you second-guessing what you're even doing. Am I a caregiver? Is this caregiving? Do I deserve to call it that? Yes, you do.

If you're regularly managing appointments, medications, routines, decision-making, or emotional support for a loved one—especially if they are chronically ill, disabled, aging, or neurodivergent—you are a caregiver. This could include tasks such as scheduling doctor's appointments, administering medications, helping with daily activities like bathing and dressing, providing emotional support, and making important decisions about their care It could also involve managing finances, coordinating with healthcare professionals, or advocating for your loved one's needs. Whether you're doing it out of love, obligation, or sheer necessity, you are holding things together that weren't yours to carry alone.

Naming your role won't make everything easier. But it does help you claim space for what you're navigating—mentally, emotionally, even spiritually. You don't have to minimize it. You don't have to earn it. You are already doing it.

The Moment You Realize Everything's Different

There isn't always a singular event that flips the switch from "family member" to "caregiver." Sometimes, it's a slow realization. Other times, it's a punch to the chest—a diagnosis, a hospitalization, or a moment when someone turns to you and says, "What should we do?"

The shift can be so subtle that it goes unnoticed. You might still be doing what you've always done—caring for someone you love—but no it includes new vocabulary, more pressure, and decisions that carry real consequences.

And that moment—that feeling of *"Oh… this is different now"*—stays with you.

Grieving What Was

One of the deepest, most invisible burdens caregivers carry is grief. Not the kind you're expected to feel after loss—but the kind that shows up before anything is gone.

It's the grief of no longer living the life you thought you would. Of watching someone you love struggle with losing spontaneity, predictability, or even the ability to plan ahead. You may grieve the loss of your job, your routines, your health, and your friendships. And sometimes, you grieve parts of yourself.

This grief is not selfish, nor is it wrong. It's a profoundly human response to the changes you're experiencing. Acknowledging this grief creates space for healing, even if that healing is as simple as catching your breath between waves of emotion.

Emotional Whiplash

Transitioning into a caregiving role often brings a mix of emotions:

Guilt: For not doing enough. Or for doing too much and resenting it.

Fear: That you'll make the wrong decision, miss a symptom, or fail your loved one.

Burnout: The slow erosion of your own energy, patience, and identity.

Grief: Not just for potential loss, but for the life you thought you would have.

These emotions are authentic and valid. They can coexist with love, hope, faith, and even joy. You don't have to choose just one. Your feelings are valid, and you are not alone in this journey.

On some days, caregiving will feel like an honor. On others, it will feel like a trap. Both can be true. It's important to remember that you are not broken because you are feeling overwhelmed. You are not weak for wishing things were different. And you are not failing just because you're tired.

A Moment I Will Never Forget – After the School Drop-Off

One day, after dropping Tre off at school, I pulled into a random parking lot and just sat in silence. My whole body felt like it had been hit by something. It wasn't a panic attack. It wasn't a breakdown. It was more like a realization that settled deep in my chest: This is my life now. Appointments. Therapies. Paperwork. Hypervigilance. IEP meetings. Meltdowns. Micro-decisions that could have ripple effects. And always being the one who had to know what to do next, even when I didn't.

I was exhausted. Not from lack of sleep, but from constant bracing. From being alert. I always anticipate what might go wrong. And no one had warned me how heavy that kind of mental and emotional labor would be.

I wasn't looking for a cure or a fix. I was looking for a moment to catch my breath. That moment became a sacred pause where I could grieve, breathe, and remember that I was still a person, not just a role.

The Caregiving Mirror – Chapter 2 Reflection Questions

When did you first realize your role had shifted?

What are you grieving that others may not see?

What emotions have been most challenging to name or accept?

Have you claimed the word "caregiver" for yourself? Why or why not?

What would it look like to make space for both grief and grace?

If you're feeling lost in your new role, you're not alone. Visit www.receptivewisdom.com for reflection tools, identity support, and guidance to help you process the grief behind caregiving.

Chapter 3
How to Speak "Doctor"

Medical Terms Made Simple and Why It Matters

One of the first and most empowering parts of caregiving is learning to understand medical language. You're suddenly surrounded by acronyms, lab results, medication instructions, and doctors who speak in shorthand. It can feel like being dropped into a foreign country without a translator—only this time, your loved one's health depends on your ability to keep up. However, as you grasp these terms, you gain a sense of control and empowerment over the situation, which makes you feel more confident and capable in your role as a caregiver.

I learned this the hard way.

When Alex was hospitalized, her doctors used terms like "DVT," "PE," and "SLE" as if I had gone to medical school. I didn't. But I asked questions, took notes, and researched everything—either online or through trusted family members with experience. Eventually, I understood that DVT stood for deep vein thrombosis, PE for pulmonary embolism, and SLE for systemic lupus erythematosus. These weren't just medical jargon; they were crucial to understanding what was happening to my daughter and how to advocate for her treatment. This understanding was not just knowledge; it was empowerment.

When Tre came to live with my husband and me, I was suddenly thrown into a different world of caregiving—one filled with assessments, psychological evaluations, developmental pediatrics, behavior therapy, and early intervention. Words like echolalia, stimming, and sensory integration were tossed around in reports. But I didn't let the language intimidate me. I took a proactive approach. I asked for definitions. I took notes. I learned. This proactive approach kept me engaged and in control of the situation, making me feel more confident in my caregiving role.

You don't need a medical degree. You need a strategy.

Understanding Medical Language: A Source of Empowerment

Medical terms aren't just words, they're tools. Tools that can unlock access to better care or build walls that shut you out.

You don't need to be fluent in medical language. But knowing how to engage with it makes a difference. It helps you:

Ask for clarification without shame!

Take notes in real time.

Spot key terms related to your loved one's condition.

Repeat what you've heard in your own words.

I recall sitting in a room while a doctor discussed "ANA titers" and "complement levels" about Alex. I had no idea what those meant. But I didn't stay in the dark. I wrote them down. Later, I looked them up and came back with questions. This process of asking questions made me feel more informed and prepared, ready to advocate for my loved one's care. Something shifted after that.

At that moment in the doctor's room was a turning point. Instead of being talked over, I was spoken to. I wasn't just the mom in the room—I became an integral part of the team. It was a powerful lesson that even a basic understanding of medical language can transform your role as a caregiver.

A Few Terms I Had to Learn the Hard Way

Ejection Fraction – How well the heart pumps blood (Mom's heart failure)

ANA (Antinuclear Antibody) – A marker for autoimmune conditions like lupus (Alex)

IEP / 504 Plan – Education terms, not medical, but vital for Tre's neurodivergent needs

Palliative vs. Hospice Care – Palliative is comfort during illness; hospice is comfort at the end of life.

One of the most helpful habits I developed was keeping a notebook to track medical terms and their meanings. This small practice not only helped me remember and understand the complex medical jargon but also gave me a sense of control and confidence in the face of uncertainty.

Practical Tips for "Speaking Doctor"

Repeat what you heard: "So what I'm hearing is…"

Ask for plain language: "Can you explain that in a way I can share with my family?"

Write things down—even if you don't understand them yet

Don't be afraid to pause: "Can we go back for a second?"

Clarify meaning: "Is that the same as…?"

Ask the Right Questions

At appointments, your goal is to understand, not impress. Try asking:

"What are the risks and benefits?"

"What happens if we wait?"

"What other options are there?"

"Can you put that in writing or send a follow-up email?"

"Is there a written treatment plan we have access to?"

Caregiver Scripts

When emotions are high and systems feel cold, these phrases can help:

"Can you explain that in simpler terms?"

"I need to make sure I understand this correctly…"

"Can we pause for a moment?"

"I want to be a partner in their care—not just a bystander."

"Can you send me a summary of today's visit?"

What to Record

You may remember it all. You won't. Keep track of:

Diagnoses and exact medical codes

Test results (especially changes over time)

Medication changes

Specialist instructions

Follow-ups and next steps

I often brought a way to take notes to medical appointments or doctor consults. More than once, this helped me clarify a detail I'd missed in the moment.

Build a Translation Toolkit

Some tools that helped me decode doctor-speak:

Medical dictionaries or apps (like MedlinePlus)

Support groups and caregiver forums

Patient portals with glossary tools

Templates I created for meds, questions, and symptoms

You can find my printable templates at www.receptivewisdom.com.

Be Confident in the Room

You belong there.

If you don't understand, ask. If something feels off, say so. If the answer doesn't sit right, get a second opinion. That's not disloyalty, it's smart caregiving. Remember, you are your loved one's best advocate. Your voice matters, and your questions and concerns are valid. Don't hesitate to speak up and ensure your loved one receives the best possible care. Trust your instincts; they are often right, and they give you the confidence to advocate effectively.

And remember: You are the expert on your loved one. Your observations and insights are invaluable.

Doctors might understand science, but you see the in-between. The symptoms they don't. The subtle changes that never make it into a chart. Your voice is not just important, it's essential.

Not Every Provider Is the Right Fit

A white coat doesn't necessarily equate to compassion. Some providers rush, dismiss, or intimidate. Trust your gut. If something doesn't feel right, you're allowed to ask for someone new. You're allowed to switch doctors.

A good provider sees your loved one—not just their diagnosis—and respects your role as part of the team.

A Personal Reminder

You are not stupid for asking questions.

You are not a burden for advocating.

You are not just a caregiver; you are an advocate, a crucial part of the care team.

And that makes you powerful.

A Moment I Will Never Forget: The Bag We Didn't Pack

The day we met Dr. Passo, I expected we'd be admitted on the spot. Alex was that sick. However, he provided us with a referral for a leg ultrasound instead. No urgency in his voice—just quiet concern.

Oddly enough, we didn't pack a bag the next day. We were at a hospital close to home. Maybe I was in denial. Perhaps I just wanted to believe one more day that she was okay.

But we didn't go home for 21 days. The scan revealed a massive blood clot. She was admitted immediately. Nine days in the PICU followed.

That day everything changed. Not just because of the diagnosis, but also because I realized something else: doctors don't always say everything. But if you learn their language, you can also hear what they're not saying.

The Caregiving Mirror – Chapter 3

What medical terms or systems have I had to learn so far?

Do I feel comfortable asking healthcare professionals for clarity?

What's one thing I want to better understand about my loved one's condition?

Helpful tools like symptom logs, appointment trackers, and medication charts are available at www.receptivewisdom.com to support you through the day-to-day details.

Chapter 4
Surviving the Administrative Avalanche

Managing Meds and Medical Paperwork Without Losing Your Mind

I never imagined how many hours of my life would be spent managing someone else's medications, insurance claims, reviewing medical records, and overseeing overall healthcare.

As a caregiver, you wear many hats-you're a support system, a pharmacist, a records clerk, an appointment coordinator, and a communicator between medical staff and the patient. Your role is not just about handing out pills, coordinating appointments, or completing endless paperwork. It's about understanding what is needed, why it's needed, when it's needed, and how or by whom you obtain what is needed. You are the one who adjusts in real time when a doctor changes the treatment plan. Your role is crucial, and your efforts are invaluable. Your adaptability in these ever-changing roles is a testament to your resilience.

Caregiving is like solving a puzzle that keeps changing shape. The administrative side of caregiving isn't just tedious; it's critical. And you're not just helping. You're managing care. You are the system holding the system together.

When it comes to managing someone's health care, a system is not just a convenience; it's a necessity. I didn't start with one. I started with a pile of papers on the kitchen counter, sticky notes on the fridge, and medication bottles scattered across the bathroom shelf. But the need for a system became clear when a pharmacist handed me the wrong dosage of my mom's diabetic medication. That moment shook me. I realized that organization isn't just about making your life easier. It's about taking control. It's about preventing harm. It's about saving lives.

That changed the day a pharmacist handed me the wrong dosage of my mom's diabetic medication—and I only caught the error because I'd jotted her dose on an index card I kept in my purse. That moment shook me. I realized that organization isn't just about making your life easier. It's about taking control. It's about preventing harm. It's about saving lives.

Having a system in place can also bring a profound sense of relief, a feeling that is often rare in this role. It may not get perfection or ease, but it does bring a little less chaos. In the world of caregiving, that's a victory. It's a comforting feeling to know that you have a structure in place, a system that can help you navigate the complexities of caregiving. This reassurance is a much-needed respite in the whirlwind of caregiving responsibilities.

And let me be honest: the fear of making a mistake is a genuine concern. It's a fear that many caregivers share, and it's okay to feel this way.

It's essential to acknowledge this fear, as it indicates that you are not alone in your concerns.

When I was managing medications for my mom, as I previously stated, I kept an index card in my wallet with her latest med list—because I knew at any moment someone might ask, especially in the ER. Later, with Alex, I had a full three-ring binder notebook containing her medications, lab test results, appointments, insurance paperwork, and other relevant information. Before the binder, I felt like I was constantly checking and rechecking, afraid that one missed detail could send everything spiraling out of control. After I created and organized the binder, caregiving was less chaotic.

With Tre, the pressure was different. Initially, it wasn't about lab results and medication dosage; it was therapies and what would work best for him. You think speech therapy, occupational therapy, or ABA therapy is one size that fits all, and once you make it to the top of the wait list for services, you are ecstatic for therapy to begin. Sadly, though, you quickly realize not all therapists are created equally, and you are back to where you started.

One of the most exhausting and often overlooked parts of caregiving is the administrative avalanche that accompanies it. From prescription refills and insurance claims to medical and therapy appointments, assessments, and insurance authorization, it's enough to overwhelm even the most organized person.

The Paper Trail No One Prepares You For

Nobody tells you that caregiving means becoming an unpaid administrator, personal assistant, and crisis coordinator—all before breakfast.

The paperwork alone can crush you: intake forms, insurance approvals, medical records, 8-32 pages of medical reports, letters of medical necessity, IEP documents, pharmacy issues, FMLA leave, billing

errors, denials, and appeals. And when you finally learn the system… it changes.

There are days you spend more time on hold than you do with the person you're caring for.

You find yourself scribbling the names of medications, checking portal logins at 2 a.m., and reserving entire sections of your brain for dates, policies, and acronyms. It's invisible labor—but labor, nonetheless.

And if you make a mistake? If a deadline is missed or a form is incomplete? You pay for it—not just in money, but in stress, care delays, or worse. It's an unforgiving system built on the assumption that you already know how to navigate it.

You didn't sign up to be an administrator. But you became one anyway. And every call, every copy, every carefully filed folder is an act of love. Even when it feels like you're drowning in paper, know this: You are doing enough, and you are doing a better job than you realize.

"I didn't go to school for this. I didn't get trained in case management or billing. But I learned—because my person needed me to. And that's what caregivers do."

Survival Tips for the Administrative Avalanche

Keep a binder or digital folder with key categories: medical, school, legal, and financial

Scan important documents and save them to a cloud drive or email

Create a simple 'In Case of Emergency' sheet with diagnoses, meds, and contact info

Ask for documentation in writing every time something is promised verbally

Designate one day a week (or even one hour) for paperwork catch-up

What Helped Me Stay Sane

Keep a Master List. Update it regularly and bring it to every appointment. Include name, dosage, purpose, prescribing doctor, and any special instructions. This list should be comprehensive, including all medications, their corresponding dosages, and the reasons for prescribing each medication. It's also essential to keep it updated with any changes in medication or dosage. Binder File. Organize it and keep it with you. Take it to every visit.

Use a Pill Organizer. It might feel old-school, but it helps prevent mistakes, especially when you're sleep-deprived. A pill organizer can help you keep track of which medications have been taken and which still need to be taken, reducing the risk of missed doses or double doses. Double-check with Pharmacists. Always ask, "Are there any interactions I should know about?" Call ahead to ensure the medication is in stock or if it needs to be ordered.

Create a 'Med Bag' for hospital trips or overnight care. Include a medication list, the names of doctors involved in the patient's medical care, a notebook, insurance cards, and a pen. Keep it near the door.

Remember, you are the one who knows your loved one best. So, don't hesitate to speak up when things feel off. Your intuition and observations are valuable in the care process.

What They Don't Tell You:

Doctors don't always talk to each other.

Pharmacy labels are sometimes unclear.

You're the only one who sees the whole picture.

You must remind each medical professional of the patient's medical history, current treatment plan, and other relevant details. EVERYTIME.

You're not 'just' helping—you're managing care. And that's no small thing.

Why Organization Matters

Staying organized helps you:

Avoid medication errors

Communicate clearly with doctors

Track symptoms over time

Handle emergencies with ease

Advocate with confidence

I've had to create systems from scratch for my mom, Alex, and Tre. Now, I want to save you that time and stress.

Start with a Medical Binder A simple 3-ring binder can become your caregiving command center. Include:

The Unintentional Caregiver

Personal Info: Name, birthdate, allergies, emergency contacts

Diagnosis History

Medication Log

Appointment Notes

Lab and Test Results

Treatment plan

Insurance Info

Legal Documents (POA, living will, HIPAA forms)

Want templates for your binder? Download them at www.receptivewisdom.com.

Manage Medications Like a Pro by Tracking the following:

Medication names (brand/generic)

Dosage and frequency

Prescribing doctor

Pharmacy used

Side effects

Start/stop dates

Tips to Stay on Top:

- Use a pill organizer
- Set alarms
- Refill early
- Call the pharmacy before you run out

Trust but Verify

Errors happen. Pharmacies mislabel. Doctors overlook interactions. Always double-check.

Digital Tools vs. Paper Systems

Use what works for you. There is no perfect method, but having a system in place helps everyone. Here are some suggestions:

- Apps: MyMeds, Medisafe, CareZone
- Google Docs/Sheets
- Patient Portals
- Paper: trackers, calendars, notebooks

I use apps for reminders but still carry a paper planner.

Prepare for the Unexpected

Keep a grab-and-go folder in the car or near the door for easy access. Include:

- Current med list
- Key diagnoses

Emergency contacts

Insurance copies

POA or consent forms

This has saved me during school meetings or medical emergencies.

Caregiving Is Hard—But This Part Can Be Easier.

You don't have to remember everything. You need a system that reminds you. Whether it's a binder, an app, or a labeled shoebox, the goal is to keep the chaos in check so you can focus on what matters: your loved one. You're already carrying so much. Let this chapter lighten the load.

A Moment I Will Never Forget – Hope from LEGOs

Before we had a diagnosis for Tre, we were living in the unknown. Tre was nonverbal. He couldn't tell us what he wanted, what he liked, or how he felt. Every day, I felt like trying to parent through a locked door.

Then, one quiet morning, Jeff and I were in the kitchen making breakfast. Tre wandered off—no prompting, no words—just his calm sense of purpose. He went to his room, found all the tiny pieces of a LEGO set—a yellow baby chick—and came back. He sat down and, without help, put the whole thing together. Piece by piece. No instructions. No assistance. Just focus.

That was the moment I knew: his mind was working deeply and beautifully. He was in there. He was following steps, thinking in order, building something from the inside out.

I didn't say it out loud, but something in me changed that day. I stopped measuring him against other kids and started watching

more closely for the ways he would show me what he understood. He didn't need words to convey his message.

And what I saw... was hope.

The Caregiving Mirror – Chapter 4

What systems or habits do I currently use to track my medications?

Where do I feel the most overwhelmed or unsure?

What would give me more confidence in managing this part of caregiving?

Paperwork can feel overwhelming, but you don't have to do it alone.

For printable tools to help you organize paperwork, track appointments, and manage care details, visit www.receptivewisdom.com and explore the free caregiver toolkit.

Chapter 5
Crisis Mode

How to Stay Calm, Be Prepared, and Get the Care Your Loved One Needs

Emergencies don't come with warning labels. One moment, you're making breakfast. Next, you're calling 911 or racing to the ER. Whether it's a sudden fall, a medication reaction, or symptoms you know aren't right, everything else fades away, and you shift into crisis mode.

I've lived through more emergency room visits than I can count—my mom's heart issues, Alex's complex medical history that warranted visits. Tre's injuries that could have typically been handled with a doctor's visit if he didn't need to be sedated for treatment. Each time, I had to learn how to walk into those chaotic rooms with a plan—even if I was falling apart inside. Here's how you can do the same.

Calm Is a Skill, not a Personality Trait

Staying calm in a crisis is not a personality trait; it's a *skill* that can *be* learned. As a caregiver, you may find yourself needing to steady your voice while your insides are in turmoil. This is not denial, it's a survival skill. Taking one breath, one step, and focusing on one task at a time can help you stay grounded when panic threatens to take over.

Quick Grounding Trick:

Look around and name:

- 5 things you can see

- 4 things you can touch

- 3 things you can hear

- 2 things you can smell

- 1 thing you can taste

This resets your brain in under a minute.

Prepare Before the Emergency

While you can't predict a crisis, you *can* certainly prepare for it. Preparation is not just a step; it's a source of power and control in the face of uncertainty. By being prepared, you can navigate the chaos of an emergency with confidence and clarity.

Emergency Folder: Keep it in a readily accessible location. Include:

- Current medication list

- Diagnoses and brief history

- Emergency contacts

- Insurance cards

- Power of attorney or consent forms

- Allergies (especially to medications)

- Preferred hospital or specialists

I had one for each of my loved ones. With Mom, it prevented medical errors. With Alex, it helped avoid delays. And with Tre, it meant I could advocate—even when others didn't understand him.

Downloadable Templates: Emergency pages and visit logs are available at www.receptivewisdom.com

Pack a Go-Bag (Don't forget to include your needs, too!)

Include:

- Emergency folder

- Phone charger and contact list

- Notebook and pen

- Comfort items (blanket, toy, headphones)

- Snacks, water, and a light jacket

Items for you- light jacket, snacks, medication, etc.

When Tre went to the ER, his headphones and favorite toy helped him cope with the situation. For Alex, I always brought her own blanket. Those small touches made a big difference.

Advocate Under Pressure

Even when you're scared, remember you are the expert on your loved one.

Speak calmly and clearly:

"My daughter has lupus and a history of blood clots. She's on a blood thinner."

"My grandson has sensory processing disorder—bright lights and loud noise overwhelm him."

"My mom has heart failure. She must stay on her med schedule."

Ask direct questions:

• What are you giving them—and why?

• What does that test show?

• When will we get the results?

• Are there any potential side effects to be aware of?

• What happens next?

Track everything

- Doctor and nurse names

- Medications and timing

- Tests ordered and results

- New symptoms or reactions

Use a notebook because stress is a thief. You won't remember everything later.

Know When to Escalate

Sometimes things go wrong. The nurse doesn't come. The doctor rushes. Your loved one is in pain. Listen to your gut. If the thought of escalating has crossed your mind you probably need to escalate.

What to do

- Politely repeat your concern: "I'm worried. Can someone check on them now?"

- Ask for the charge nurse

- Request patient advocacy or a supervisor if needed

You're not being rude. You're being firm. I've had to use my assertive voice more than I should, but it's part of the job. Don't be afraid to use it; your loved one is counting on you.

The Emotional Aftermath

The emotional crash after a crisis is real—fatigue, fog, guilt, grief. It's okay to feel this way. Let yourself feel it and know that you're not alone in this. The emotional aftermath of a crisis is a natural part of the caregiving journey, and it's essential to acknowledge and process these feelings.

Then:

- Review and organize your notes
- Update your medical binder
- Schedule follow-ups or referrals
- Rest—even briefly

You can't pour from an empty cup. You matter, too.

Crisis Checklist for Caregivers

What to Bring:

- ID and insurance cards
- Medication list (with dosages and timing)
- Diagnoses, allergies, and surgery history
- POA or health directives

Comfort Items:

- Phone charger
- Snacks, water
- Blanket, lip balm, sensory item

Questions to Ask Providers:

- What are we ruling out with this test?

- What does this diagnosis mean short-term and long-term?

- What should I watch for after discharge?

- Who do I call if symptoms worsen?

Bonus Tip: Keep a *Go Folder* (digital or physical) ready. It'll save you precious time and stress when minutes matter most.

You don't have to be fearless. You need to be prepared—and that's a kind of strength, too.

A Moment I Will Never Forget – The Scan That Saved Her Life

Several days into Alex's hospital stay, her breathing worsened. Despite treatment for blood clots, she wasn't improving. A new CT scan was ordered. Her specialist, Dr. Passo, was hours away and reviewed it remotely. He said it looked fine. But a few days later, while in town for a speaking engagement, he stopped by the hospital on instinct.

Thank God he did.

What hadn't been visible digitally was clear in person: Alex was bleeding internally. The medication meant to save her was causing her lungs to hemorrhage.

He told us later: her lungs looked "like a colander—just pouring blood." She was moved to the PICU and began emergency treatment. That visit saved her life.

I believe God tapped into Dr. Passo's intuition that day. It was a divine appointment—one I will never forget.

The Caregiving Mirror – Chapter 5

Do I have an emergency plan in place?

What would I want in my hands if I had to rush out the door?

How do I stay grounded during a medical crisis?

What steps could I take to prepare for the next unexpected moment?

In urgent moments, having the right tools nearby can bring peace of mind.

Visit www.receptivewisdom.com for helpful and supportive tools and resources for emergency situations

Chapter 6
Navigating Systems That Are Supposed to Help

Insurance, Schools, Government Agencies, Advocating with Paperwork, Patience and Grit.

As if caregiving wasn't hard enough, now you're faced with a mountain of paperwork, endless phone calls, and systems so convoluted they seem designed to test your patience. Another challenging aspect of caregiving isn't the care itself but instead dealing with the systems that are supposed to help.

Healthcare. Insurance. Special education. Social Security. Medicaid. Case management. These are not just separate entities, but a complex web of systems that you, as a caregiver, are expected to navigate. The intricacies of these systems can be overwhelming, but with the right strategies, you can successfully navigate them.

These systems exist to offer support, but too often, they're confusing, slow, and impersonal. You'd think once someone is diagnosed, there would be a clear path forward. But instead, you're handed a few brochures,

a list of referrals, and a stack of paperwork. No one says, "Here's what this means and what to do next." I had to figure it out the hard way—usually during a crisis.

With my mother, I spent countless hours on the phone with insurance companies, trying to decipher what was covered and what wasn't. Her medications were far from affordable, and every prescription felt like a battle. One person would say yes, another would say no. Forms were misplaced, and approvals were delayed. I quickly learned that it wasn't just about submitting—you had to follow up, call back, ask for names, and sometimes, even ask for supervisors.

With Tre, it was another world—early intervention service, therapies, special education law, disability benefits. I had to learn about IEPs, how to request evaluations, and what accommodations are allowed under a 504 Plan. Every agency has its own rules. Every state is different. And no one gives you a cheat sheet.

This chapter is here to help you find your footing in the middle of all that.

When the System Feels Like the Enemy

There were days I cried—not because of the diagnosis, but because of the red tape. It's exhausting to continually prove that your loved one needs

help, begging for services that should be basic. To feel invisible in a room full of professionals.

But here's what I learned: persistence pays off. You may not win every battle, but your voice builds something—momentum, credibility, a paper trail. Over time, that matters. It's not about winning every time, but about the journey and the progress you make along the way. Your persistence is your power, and it's what keeps you moving forward.

Remember, every step you take in navigating these systems is a step towards better care for your loved one.

What No One Tells You

You may have to apply more than once. Denials are common.

Documentation is everything. Keep a folder. Print emails. Take notes.

You'll repeat your story to intake workers, case managers, and school teams.

There is no central coordinator. You are the case manager now.

Staff change constantly, including the therapist you grow fond of.

What Helped Me Stay Sane

Start a simple binder or digital folder.

Break it into categories: medical, benefits, school, therapy.

Keep a running timeline.

Document key dates—diagnoses, applications, approvals, denials, evaluations. It will save you later.

Use go-to phrases when calling:

"I'm following up on a request submitted on [date]."

"Can you confirm your name and a direct line in case we're disconnected?"

"Is there another benefit or service we may qualify for that hasn't been mentioned yet?"

That last one led me to resources I didn't even know existed.

Start with Documentation

Regardless of the system, documentation is your power tool. Save everything:

Letters and notices

Test results

Diagnoses and evaluations

Treatment plans

IEP or 504 Plans

Appeals and denials

When Alex was denied critical medication, I used her records to file a successful appeal. When Tre needed more school support, paperwork from therapists made our case undeniable.

Understanding Insurance (Even When It Makes No Sense)

You'll hear terms like "not medically necessary," "out of network," or "needs prior authorization."

How to survive it:

Document every call: date, time, name, summary

Ask for denials in writing

Ask why it was denied

Keep track of renewal dates and required authorizations

Learn your rights—every state has a Department of Insurance

When Mom's heart meds were denied, I filed a grievance with help from her doctor, and we won. It was a fight. But it worked.

Special Education and the School System

When Tre entered school, I saw how difficult it was to get services, even with a precise diagnosis.

Tips:

Request evaluations in writing

Understand the difference between an IEP and a 504 Plan

Attend meetings and take notes

Bring support if needed

Ask for prior written notice after decisions are made

When the principal at Tre's school wanted to reduce the school day to two hours, knowing his civil rights was what won that battle. Yes, there will be battles you will fight that you won't imagine until they happen.

Government Programs: SSI, Medicaid, Case Management

These applications are time-consuming and detail-heavy. Don't go in unprepared.

Start early

Be honest about limitations (don't minimize them)

Keep a copy of everything

Follow up—repeatedly

Submit as much documentation as possible upfront

I applied for Tre once and had approval within four months. It's possible—with preparation.

Case Managers and Advocates

Some are amazing. Some aren't. Ask yourself:

Do they listen?

Do they follow through?

Do they explain things clearly?

Do they return your calls?

If not, you can request someone new. I've done it more than once. Remember, you're not alone in this. Some people can offer assistance, and it's perfectly fine to ask for it. It's not a sign of weakness, but a sign of strength and determination. Seeking help is not a sign of defeat; it's a sign that you're not alone in this journey.

Don't Take "No" as the Final Answer

Appeals aren't a last resort—they're part of the process. You can appeal:

Insurance denials

School decisions

Service rejections

Benefit determinations

Persistence is your leverage

What I Wish I'd Known

Don't wait for the system to offer help. Ask. Document. Repeat.

Professionals may care, but they're overloaded. You still need to follow up.

You don't need to be perfect. You need to keep showing up.

Red Flags and Roadblocks

When the system breaks down, it can look like this:

You get conflicting answers from different staff members

Your paperwork is "lost" more than once

You're discouraged from asking questions

Pressure tactics are used to force decisions

No one seems to know who's in charge of your case

You're always following up with no clear direction

You're not imagining it. These are signs of a broken system—and it's not your fault.

What You Can Do

Keep a log (names, times, conversations)

Follow up in writing

Ask for things in plain language

Request a supervisor or advocate

Use a tracker or app to stay on top of deadlines

You don't have to know everything. You just must be persistent. And remember—your purpose is powerful.

"Systems may be slow, but I've learned to be louder, steadier, and more prepared. They have policies, but I have a purpose, and sometimes exceptions to policies are warranted."

You Are Not Powerless.

You are not small.

You are not invisible.

You're a fierce advocate—and that counts.

You've already done something most people haven't: fought for someone's survival. You can fight through the systems, too.

A Moment I Will Never Forget – *Learning Still Found Us*

When Alex was too sick for school, I feared she would fall behind—not just academically, but emotionally as well. Her world had already shrunk so much.

But then her homebound teacher arrived—my mother-in-law. A seasoned educator with a gentle spirit, she filled our home with more than math lessons. She brought peace, grace, and a return to normalcy.

They weren't just reviewing assignments. They were preserving hope—one worksheet at a time.

Even when systems fail, sometimes the right people show up. Learning doesn't always happen in a classroom. Sometimes, it happens at the kitchen table, surrounded by love.

The Caregiving Mirror – Chapter 6

What systems (insurance, education, government programs) have I interacted with as a caregiver, and what was that experience like?

Where have I felt most overwhelmed or unsupported by "the system"? How did I respond?

What strategies have helped me stay organized through all the paperwork, deadlines, and follow-ups?

Who can I ask for help when I feel lost in the red tape?

What advocacy win (big or small) am I proud of?

How can I remind myself that persistence is a powerful force, even when progress feels slow?

Stay organized with downloadable tools like visit summaries, system logs, and contact trackers at www.receptivewisdom.com — created to help you advocate clearly and confidently.

Chapter 7
The Pivot That Changes the Journey

Moments of clarity that shift you from reaction to advocacy

There's a moment in caregiving when something finally clicks. It doesn't always come with clarity or closure, but something shifts. The fog lifts just enough to see what has been in front of you all along. And even if no one else notices it, you do.

It's not loud. There's no music swelling in the background. Sometimes, the moment is so quiet that it barely registers—until your chest tightens, your breath catches, and your spirit whispers, *'This means something.'*

Perhaps it's the day a name is finally given to what you've been witnessing and worrying over. A diagnosis that doesn't fix things but explains them. A set of words that validates the sleepless nights, the unanswered questions, the instinct that something wasn't quite right. This moment brings a profound sense of relief, a validation of your concerns, and a clear direction for the journey ahead. It's a reassurance that you're not alone in this, that others see what you see, and that there's a path forward.

Or it's not a diagnosis at all.

It could be something smaller, but no less sacred. A glance held a second longer. A word spoken after months of silence. A gentle nod from a loved one who usually turns away. These small, meaningful moments are like beacons of hope, reminding you that something, anything, is connecting.

Sometimes, it's the moment someone else—someone in a position of power—finally listens. A doctor who stops rushing. A teacher who shifts their tone. A caseworker who finally sees your child or your parent as a person, not a file. These are the moments that empower you, that give you the confidence to advocate for your loved one. They remind you that you have a voice, that your concerns are valid, and that you can make a difference in the care your loved one receives.

These are the moments that don't make headlines.

But they crack something open.

They remind you why you keep going.

Whatever it is, that moment lands deep in your bones.

Not because everything is solved—but because, for the first time, you're not the only one who sees it.

You're not alone in the knowing.

And that changes everything.

Before the Answers Come

And yet, before that moment arrives, there's a stretch of caregiving that feels like you're stumbling through the dark, emotionally and physically exhausted, and often feeling alone in your journey.

Before the answers came, I lived in a place of constant uncertainty. Every day felt like detective work with no clues to follow. That period—between the first concern and final confirmation—was its own kind of grief. If you're still in that place, you're not forgotten. This chapter is also for you, to remind you of the importance of acknowledging and processing your emotions. It's okay to feel the weight of the unknown, to grieve the loss of the life you once knew, and to seek support in these moments. You're not alone in this journey of caregiving.

The Day Everything Shifts

When Alex was diagnosed with systemic lupus erythematosus (SLE) at 14, I felt like the ground dropped out from under me. We had spent months in and out of hospitals, piecing together strange and frightening symptoms—joint pain, blood clots, fevers, chest pain—and now we finally had a name for it. But knowing didn't make it easier. It made it more real.

Later, when Tre was diagnosed, I had a similar mix of emotions. On the one hand, I was relieved. I finally had documentation to support what I knew deep down: that his development wasn't typical, and he needed support. On the other hand, I grieved. Not because I didn't love him exactly as he was, but because I knew the road ahead would be long, complicated, and unfair.

The Unintentional Caregiver

When Tre received his diagnosis, it didn't fix everything. But it gave me language. It gave me tools. And more than anything, it gave me the ability to step into advocacy mode.

Before that, I'd wondered: Was I doing something wrong? Was I missing something obvious? Was he okay, and I didn't know how to parent him? After the diagnosis, I could finally answer: No. I wasn't failing. I loved a child who needed different support. And I could start learning what that looked like.

For Alex, the answers came in pieces. Lupus is complicated. Her symptoms didn't always line up with the lab results. But each time we found a medication that helped, a specialist who listened, or a moment when she said, "I feel better today," it felt like a small victory. Those answers didn't solve everything, but they gave us direction.

With Mom, things were more gradual. Her health declined over the years, and new diagnoses kept coming—congestive heart failure, diabetes, neuropathy, and vascular issues. There wasn't a single diagnosis moment, but rather a slow accumulation of conditions that gradually took more and more of her independence. This journey requires patience and resilience, and you are not alone in this.

Each diagnosis was different, but each one changed my life.

Getting answers doesn't mean the journey is over. It just means you can stop circling the same questions in the dark. You can start making decisions. You can start breathing a little easier.

You'll still have hard days. But now you're walking with a flashlight—and that changes everything.

When Everything Changes Overnight

There's a particular kind of heartbreak that happens when a healthy child—one who ran through the yard last week or aced a math test yesterday—is suddenly extremely sick.

You go from everyday life to emergency rooms in a matter of days. From planning birthday parties to learning how to pronounce the names of medications you've never heard before. From grocery lists to surgery prep. From soccer games to PICU monitors.

No one prepares you for that kind of whiplash

When Alex got sick, it felt as though the entire world had tilted. We weren't gradually introduced to her illness. There was no gentle warning. Just a string of frightening symptoms, a few urgent doctor visits, and then… a diagnosis that changed everything.

She didn't look sick at first. That made it harder. Even as we juggled hospital stays, chemo, and side effects, people would say, "But she looks fine." What they didn't see were the fevers that came without warning. The clots. The medications have names longer than most words in the dictionary. The constant fear.

For parents, the toll is indescribable. You become a medical researcher overnight. You don't sleep. You hold your breath through every lab result. You brace yourself for the worst and still hope for the best. You put your pain on a shelf so you can be strong for your child. It's okay to feel overwhelmed; it's perfectly normal to carry the weight of this journey. You are not alone in this.

But it doesn't stop there.

Siblings feel it, too. They watch their brother or sister get all the attention—because they have to—and wonder where that leaves them.

They act out or shut down. They worry silently. They carry their own guilt, fear, and confusion in ways they don't yet know how to express.

The whole family changes

Routines disappear. Financial strain mounts. Jobs may be lost or reshuffled. Relationships are tested. Time becomes measured in blood draws and scan results instead of calendar events.

And through it all, caregivers try to hold everything together.

If you're in the midst of this right now, I want to say this clearly: you're not failing. You're surviving something unimaginable.

Give yourself credit for showing up—for every question you've asked, every medication you've administered, every meltdown you've weathered, every decision you've made on limited sleep and unlimited love.

"The day everything changed was the day I learned just how deep love runs—deeper than sleep, deeper than fear, deeper than anyone on the outside will ever understand."

You're Allowed to Feel Everything

When the answers finally come, they can bring a tidal wave of emotion.

There's no "right" way to respond to a diagnosis. You might feel:

Numb

Angry

Relieved

Grief-stricken

Guilty

Hopeful

Exhausted

Sometimes, you'll feel all of them at once. And that's okay.

Let yourself process. Cry in the car. Yell into a pillow. Journal. Call a friend. Take a walk. Sit in silence. Do whatever helps you start to move through the shock.

Caregivers often skip this part. We jump straight into problem-solving. But the emotional weight doesn't dissipate simply because you're busy. Give yourself room to feel.

Gather Your Team

After the diagnosis, you'll likely be thrown into a whirlwind of new appointments, tests, and specialists.

Start building your support system—medical and otherwise.

Medical Team:

Primary care doctor or pediatrician

Specialists (rheumatologist, neurologist, developmental pediatrician)

Pharmacist

Support Team:

Therapist (for your loved one and maybe yourself)

Peer caregivers and local groups

Admin Team:

Case manager or social worker

IEP or education plan coordinator

Start with one or two people you trust and build from there.

Learn—But Don't Drown in Information

When Alex was diagnosed with lupus, I stayed up all night reading medical journals, blog posts, and treatment guidelines. I wanted to know everything. But I also scared myself.

Eventually, I learned to strike a balance. What helped:

Use reliable sources (hospital websites, nonprofits, medical associations)

Join support groups—but don't let every story sink you

Ask your providers for trusted resources

With Tre, I learned to pace myself. There was no rush. What mattered most was showing up, asking questions, and trusting our process.

What to Say When You Don't Know What to Say

Here are a few phrases that helped me:

"We just got the diagnosis and are still learning."

"We're focused on building a care plan."

"I don't have all the words, but I'm here and I care."

Next Steps: Planning and Advocating

Start small, then build a long-term plan.

Begin with:

Medications or treatments

Therapy referrals

Paperwork deadlines

Emotional support

Then ask:

What does ongoing care look like?

Are there any financial considerations?

What supports do we need?

Start asking early:

What does this diagnosis mean day-to-day?

What treatment options exist?

What support is available?

What are our rights?

Advocacy is part of caregiving now. Embrace it with confidence and care.

You're Still the Same—But Everything Has Changed

Give yourself grace. You're navigating the unknown with courage and love. You won't always get it right. But if you keep showing up, keep learning, and keep loving, you're doing enough.

Let This Be Your Turning Point

A diagnosis may feel like an ending.

But it's also a beginning shift into healing, learning, and growth. This is the day the answers come.

Maybe not all of them. Maybe not perfectly.

But enough to take the next step.

You're not alone. I've walked this path. And I'll keep walking with you.

If You're Still Waiting for Answers

Keep asking. Keep showing up. Keep trusting what you see—especially if others don't yet.

You're not crazy. You're not overreacting.

You are not alone.

A Moment I Will Never Forget – Advocacy Preserving Joy

Near the end of her senior year, Alex was taking blood thinners and undergoing regular lab tests. One day, her results came back dangerously off. The doctor warned her not to drive or even leave the house. But something felt off.

She had no symptoms. I asked for a retest. They refused.

So I took her myself, using her standing lab order. The new results? Normal.

That quiet moment—driving to the lab, trusting my instinct—preserved her joy, her graduation, and a piece of her independence.

What I didn't say out loud was how close we came to losing everything because of one error and one refusal to listen. But I knew. And I'll never forget.

The Caregiving Mirror – Chapter 7

What answer changed everything for me, even in a small way?

How did I feel when someone finally understood what I was trying to say?

When the dust settles after a diagnosis, clarity becomes your greatest tool. Visit www.receptivewisdom.com for planning templates and reflection prompts designed to help you take the next step with confidence.

Chapter 8
Planning for the Future
Legal, Financial, and End-of-Life

Facing Hard Topics with Clarity, Love, and Strength

I never wanted to become an expert in civil rights law. I just wanted to protect my grandson.

When Tre was physically assaulted by a contractor working with him at school, I was heartbroken—and furious. The contractor's actions left Tre with a broken arm and severe emotional trauma. What made it worse was what the school attempted afterward: they tried to reassign the same contractor to another student and cut Tre's hours down to just two per day. They were violating his rights. And they hoped I wouldn't notice.

But I did. I called for a meeting with the school administration, including the school board, to discuss Tre's situation and the need for a revised Individualized Education Program (IEP). I presented evidence of the contractor's assault and its impact on Tre's well-being. The revised

plan, which included increased security measures and a different contractor, came through the next morning.

Months later, Dr. Morris, the school principal, pulled me aside and said, "Tre is lucky to have you. Every child doesn't have a strong advocate to speak up for them." That moment reminded me that advocacy, regardless of how exhausting it is, can change outcomes. It was empowering to know my persistence made a real difference in Tre's life—and it can do the same for you and your loved one, giving you a sense of strength and capability.

That experience taught me something essential: planning isn't about paranoia—it's about protection. And it's not just for "someday." It's for the moment when things go wrong, and you need to respond with power instead of panicking. Having a plan in place can bring a sense of relief, knowing that you're prepared for whatever may come, and it can make you feel reassured and prepared.

Start with the Basics: Legal Documents Every Caregiver Should Know

Whether your loved one is young or old, aware or unable to advocate for themselves, specific legal tools can bring peace of mind—and authority—when it matters most.

Here are the essentials:

Power of Attorney (POA): Grants legal authority to act on someone's behalf—financially, medically, or both.

Healthcare Proxy: Allows you to make medical decisions on behalf of your loved one if they are unable to speak for themselves.

Living Will: Outlines preferences for life-sustaining treatment.

Will or Trust: Dictates what happens with assets and dependents. A Trust can help avoid probate and preserve eligibility for benefits.

Guardianship or Conservatorship: This may be necessary if your loved one is unable to make decisions on their own behalf due to a legal incapacity.

Note: Laws vary by state. Consult a special needs or elder law attorney for guidance.

When Alex turned 18, I had her sign a healthcare Power of Attorney (POA) so I could continue managing her care. With Tre, I've begun researching guardianship to prepare for his transition to adulthood. This process involves understanding his rights and responsibilities, as well as the legal implications of his decisions. And with my mom, I had to make decisions without any roadmap, because we hadn't planned far enough ahead.

Learn from me. Don't wait.

Financial Planning: A Necessity for All Caregivers. Caregiving has a profound impact on every aspect of your financial life. It's not just about saving money, it's about ensuring sustainability.

Start by exploring:

Caregiving impacts every part of your financial life. It's not just about savings—it's about sustainability. Start by exploring:

SSI or SSDI: Disability benefits that help cover essentials.

Medicaid and Medicare: Learn what each program covers.

Special Needs Trusts: These trusts enable a disabled loved one to receive gifts or inheritances without jeopardizing government benefits, provided they are established correctly. Seek an attorney experienced in Special Needs Trust funds.

ABLE Accounts: Tax-advantaged savings accounts for disability-related expenses.

Life Insurance: If something happens to you, what happens to your loved one?

Keep a backup: store copies of legal and financial records in both digital and physical formats.

I wish someone had told me that planning doesn't mean expecting the worst; it means protecting the people you love.

Don't Wait to Talk About End-of-Life Wishes

Whether your loved one is 25 or 85, ask:

What kind of care would you want if you couldn't speak for yourself?

Are there treatments you'd refuse?

Who should make medical decisions on your behalf?

I had this conversation with my mom in the hospital. When I asked what she wanted if she stopped breathing, she quietly said, "Let me go." It was heartbreaking, but when the moment came, I knew I was honoring her wishes. And that gave me peace.

Please put it in writing. Use living wills and advance directives to formalize your wishes.

Future Planning Checklist for Caregivers

You don't have to do it all at once. Start with one thing a week. Protecting your loved one doesn't require perfection; it just takes progress.

Legal

Durable Power of Attorney (financial decisions)

Healthcare Power of Attorney / Medical Proxy

Living Will or Advance Directive

Guardianship or custodial paperwork (if applicable)

Will or Trust documents

Financial

List of bank accounts, pensions, assets, and debts

Monthly caregiving/household budget

Insurance policies (life, health, long-term care)

Medicaid/SSI/benefits documentation

Medical & Emergency

Medication list with dosages and refill schedule

Contact information for all providers and specialists

Copies of diagnoses, test results, and discharge summaries

Emergency Plan: Who Steps In If You're Unavailable?

End-of-Life

Preferred care setting (home, hospice, facility)

Burial or cremation preferences

Obituary or service wishes (if known)

Legacy items (memory books, letters, videos, etc.)

Future planning isn't about giving up—it's about giving those you love one last act of protection and peace.

Plan for Your Own Future, Too

Ask yourself:

Who will take over if I am unable to continue caregiving?

Do I have a will and healthcare power of attorney?

Am I protected financially if I need to take a leave of absence from work?

Am I taking care of myself while caring for others?

You Matter, Too: The Importance of Self-Care Remember, taking care of yourself is not a luxury; it's a necessity. Your well-being is crucial in the caregiving journey. You are essential, and your health and happiness matter.

Final Thoughts

Planning ahead isn't about fear; it's about love. It's about knowing that when life shifts unexpectedly, you won't scramble.

You'll respond with clarity, compassion, and a plan.

Start where you are. Ask for help. You don't have to do this alone.

A Moment I Will Never Forget – Paving the Way

The first day I dropped Tre off at school after homeschooling him for over two years, my heart was in my throat.

He'd been through more than any child should—assaulted at a daycare while nonverbal. For years, schools meant fear. I promised him that when he went back, it would be different.

And it was—because I made sure of it.

I fought to have a registered behavior technician accompany him, not one assigned by the district, but one approved through our private insurance. That distinction protected him. It had never been done in our district before, but I refused to take no for an answer.

The day it was approved, I cried—not just for Tre—but for the kids who'd come after him. We changed something. We created a path.

That's advocacy. That's a legacy.

The Caregiving Mirror – Chapter 8

What legal or financial documents do I already have in place?

Have I clearly communicated my loved one's (or my own) care preferences?

What steps can I take this week to build future stability?

Do I have a way to keep all our critical records organized and accessible?

What emotions come up when I think about end-of-life planning?

Who can I talk to for legal, financial, or emotional support?

What would peace of mind look like for me, and how can I take one step closer?

Find helpful checklists and practical tools for future care planning at www.receptivewisdom.com.

Chapter 9
Building a Support Network (Even If You're Alone)

Why You Can't (and Shouldn't) Do This Alone

Caregiving often starts as a one-person mission. You step in because someone has to. You rearrange your schedule, drop your plans, and figure it out as you go. In the early days, you might not even realize how much support you'll eventually need.

But here's the truth: You can't sustain this alone. And more importantly, you don't have to.

Whether you have a full circle of family and friends or you're doing this with no one else to lean on, there are ways to build the support network you need. This process is not just about finding help; it's about empowerment. It puts you in control and boosts your confidence in your caregiving journey.

As caregivers, we're told to ask for help. But no one really prepares us for how complicated that can be. Sometimes, the help doesn't show up.

Sometimes, the help isn't helpful. And sometimes, the help makes more work for you.

Yet, we persist in our search. Because when you finally find someone who understands—someone who lightens the load instead of adding to it—it can transform your entire caregiving experience, bringing a sense of relief and comfort. This persistence is a testament to your determination and a source of hope.

You Are Allowed to Be Picky.

It's not about being difficult, it's about being discerning. You have the right to choose the best fit for your family.

When we first tried to get respite help for Tre, I was nervous. Letting someone into your home, into your child's routine, into your carefully constructed world—it's a vulnerable act. The first few caregivers didn't work out. One showed up late and didn't seem to understand sensory issues. Another was canceled twice in the first week.

But eventually, we found someone who clicked with him. She moved slowly, used soft language, and never forced a response. She didn't try to "fix" him; she just met him where he was. That was the moment I understood: you don't need perfect help, just the right fit for your family.

It took time—and lots of trial and error—to build a team. Sometimes, you have to rebuild it with little to no notice. And that's okay.

What Help Looks Like (and What It Doesn't)

Help is not:

Someone who causes more stress than relief

Someone you must constantly supervise

Someone who dismisses your instincts or minimizes your loved one's experience

Help is:

Someone who shows up

Someone who listens and adapts

Someone who treats your loved one with dignity

Advocate without apology!

Trust your gut: If someone doesn't feel like the right fit, it's okay to move on.

Ask specific questions: "How have you worked with someone with an X diagnosis before?" or "What would you do if XYZ happens?"

Establishing boundaries early on is empowering. Clearly communicate what is acceptable and what is not. Put it in writing if needed. This will help you feel secure and in charge of your caregiving journey.

Documenting everything, especially when using Medicaid or private agencies, is crucial. It enables you to stay organized and prepared, ensuring you have all the necessary information readily available.

When Help Isn't Available

There were seasons when no help came. We were on waitlists. We were denied services. We were stretched beyond capacity.

During those times, I had to redefine "help." It became:

A neighbor is bringing a meal

A friend texting to check in

My husband is taking the night shift, so I can sleep

Help doesn't always come in the form of a badge or a clipboard. Sometimes, it manifests in subtle, quiet ways. And those count, too.

The Myth of the "Strong" Caregiver

People often refer to caregivers as "strong," as if it's a compliment.

But true strength is knowing when to ask for help—and being brave enough to accept it. I used to wear independence-like armor. Eventually, I broke down. I was exhausted and barely holding things together.

That's when I learned that asking for help isn't a sign of weakness, it's a sign of survival.

Start Where You Are

Support doesn't always look like a team with casseroles and color-coded calendars. Sometimes, it's:

One person checking in

A professional you trust

A stranger in an online group who gets it

The Unintentional Caregiver

Places to Start:

Family and friends

Support groups

Neighbors and community

Medical and school professionals

Online caregiving forums

How to Sustain Support

Schedule regular check-ins

Rotate helpers to avoid burning out

Express appreciation

How to Ask for Help (Even If It's Hard)

People who want to help need direction.

Sample Script:

"Hey, I'm really stretched. Could you drop off dinner on Thursday or watch Tre for an hour while I nap?"

Tips:

Be specific

Keep a task list

Use tools like Lots of Helping Hands

Don't apologize

What to Do If You Really Are Alone

Sometimes support just isn't there. Here's what helped:

Therapy

Faith communities

Local agencies

Professional respite care

You're not failing. You're doing the work of ten people. And you still deserve support.

Boundaries Are Support, Too

It's okay to say:

"No, that won't work for us."

"Thanks, but I need something different."

"Please talk to me, not about me."

Celebrating the Good Ones

When someone truly helps, let them know. Connection is what keeps caregivers going. You may be the primary caregiver, but you don't have to hold everything alone.

Support doesn't just make caregiving easier. It makes it *possible*.

What I Didn't Say Out Loud – When Professional Help Crossed the Line

Tre was overstimulated and distressed. He wanted his comfort toy and to come to me.

The BCBA blocked both, saying he needed to learn independence.

I didn't see a strategy. I saw my child being denied comfort.

So, I emailed her supervisor and asked for her removal.

Calm. Direct. Done.

What didn't I say out loud?

Those instincts, especially caregiver instincts, move faster than exhaustion.

And credentials don't outrank compassion.

A Moment I Will Never Forget – The Right Person Finally

When I was searching for respite care for Tre, I felt like Goldilocks. Too loud. Too forceful. Too unreliable.

Provider after provider just didn't fit—not because they were bad, but because they didn't see him.

Then she showed up. Quiet voice. Gentle presence. She sat nearby and waited. He didn't flinch. He didn't shut down. He stayed.

Over time, she earned his trust. She didn't try to change him. She adapted to him.

She listened when I explained his needs.

What didn't I say out loud?

How emotional I felt watching them together.

How powerful it was to have someone walk with me, even for an hour.

After so many "almosts," we had found our yes.

I'll never forget the relief of that day.

The sigh I didn't know I was holding.

The shift from surviving to exhaling.

The Caregiving Mirror – Chapter 9

What kind of help have I found most valuable so far?

Where am I still trying to do it all alone—and why?

What's one boundary or expectation I could set more clearly?

Find support system tools and caregiver planners at www.receptivewisdom.com — because no one should have to do this alone.

Chapter 10
Taking Care of Yourself Without Guilt

Why You Matter, Too

Your self-care is not a luxury; it's a necessity.

It's a testament to your value and significance in this journey of caregiving.

Caregiving can consume your world. From sunup to well past sundown, you're doing everything for someone else—managing medications, coordinating appointments, cooking meals, calming meltdowns, researching treatments, filing paperwork, driving across town, fighting with insurance companies, and still trying to smile at the end of the day.

However, remember that, amidst all this, your own well-being is equally important.

If you're not careful, you disappear.

There's a difference between being tired and being gone.

The Unintentional Caregiver

Tired is, "I need a nap."

Gone is "I can't feel anything anymore."

I've been there—so focused on Alex's flares, Mom's declining heart, or Tre's IEP battles that I didn't realize I hadn't eaten, hadn't slept, hadn't called a friend in weeks. My needs weren't just on the back burner—they were off the stove entirely.

And if you've been caregiving long enough, you know what I mean. I've had days where I was so burned out, I forgot what I liked. I couldn't name the last time I laughed. I didn't want to talk. I just wanted everything to stop—for five minutes, an hour, a week.

It's okay to feel this way. It's a shared experience.

You're not alone in this. But here's the truth:

That's not sustainable. And it's not selfless. It's dangerous.

You cannot give what you no longer have. Your energy, clarity, and presence—your you-ness—are essential parts of the care you provide.

Burnout Doesn't Always Look Like Falling Apart

Sometimes, it looks like:

Snapping at someone you love, then feeling ashamed

Crying while folding laundry because no one notices what you carry.

Fantasizing about running away—not because you don't care, but because you care too much.

Feeling numb, flat, or resentful—even toward the person you're caring for.

You don't have to wait for a full breakdown to take burnout seriously.

The early signs matter.

Rethinking Balance

Caregiver balance isn't about spa days or weekend retreats. It's about adjusting the weight just enough to keep moving without losing yourself completely.

Balance might look like:

Saying "no" to a non-essential appointment

Letting your loved one watch an extra episode while you sit in the quiet

Choosing a frozen pizza over a home-cooked meal

Allowing the laundry to wait so you can breathe.

That's not laziness. That's wisdom.

The Guilt Trap

Guilt shows up constantly in caregiving:

"I should be doing more."

"I'm so tired, but I can't stop."

"Other people have it worse."

"If I take a break, I'm selfish."

But here's the truth:

You are allowed to need care, too.

Guilt tells you your pain doesn't matter. It urges you to keep going until you can no longer continue.

But you're not a machine.

You're a human being doing superhuman things, and even superheroes need rest.

Micro-Moments of Self-Care

You may not be able to take a vacation, but you can take a breath.

Start small. Try just 10 minutes a day:

Step outside for fresh air.

Listen to your favorite song.

Drink water and eat something nourishing.

Breathe deeply.

Text a friend who gets it

Say no to something that drains you.

These aren't luxuries. They're survival tools.

Set Boundaries (Yes, Even Now)

One of the hardest lessons I had to learn: boundaries aren't barriers. They're protection.

Say no when:

You're being asked to do more than you can carry.

Someone dismisses your needs or your loved one's.

A system demands more than it gives.

Say yes to:

Respite programs

Counseling or peer support

Help, even if it's imperfect.

Saying, "I can't do that right now," without explanation.

Boundaries aren't a weakness. They are wisdom in motion.

What Helped Me Reclaim Myself

Permission to feel everything. You can love someone and still feel trapped. You can be grateful and furious at the same time.

Finding a pocket of time that's mine. Five minutes in the car. Music while folding laundry. It didn't have to be big—it just had to be mine.

Letting go of being the only one. Even imperfect help is still help. Delegating wasn't failure, it was relief.

Telling the truth to one safe person. "I'm not okay." Those three words connected me to compassion—and reminded me I wasn't alone.

You're Still a Person

Caregiving can blur your identity. But you're still in there.

And you matter.

You are allowed to rest.

You are allowed to want joy.

You are allowed to protect your energy without apology.

Build Your "You" List

Create a list of what brings you comfort and calm, not what you *should* do, but what helps you feel like yourself.

Here's what mine looked like:

Prayer—talking with God.

Watching birds outside my dining room table.

Planting a flower garden

Coffee and silence

Music on hard days

Laughing with an old friend

Keep this list visible. When you feel lost in the role of caregiver, take it on. Choose just one thing.

Don't Wait for a Crisis

Most caregivers wait until they collapse before asking for help. I've done it. More than once. But now I know, asking for help is not a failure. It's an act of love.

Say yes to:

Meals dropped off.

A sibling taking a shift.

A stranger holding space in an online support group.

Let yourself be helped. You're not a burden.

You're a person doing something brave and brave people need backup.

You Are Worth Caring For.

Let me say this plainly:

You are more than a caregiver.

You are more than your to-do list.

You are allowed to rest, to laugh, to grieve, to dream.

You are allowed to not be okay.

You are allowed to ask for more.

And you are worth every ounce of care, compassion, and protection that you give to others.

Don't wait for someone else to give you permission.

Take it. Reclaim it. Claim yourself.

You matter, caregiver.

You always have.

Reclaiming Yourself

Caregiving has a way of shrinking your world until there's hardly any room left for the person you used to be. One day you realize you haven't read a book for pleasure in months. Or made your favorite meal. Or put on earrings.

That last one hit me harder than I expected.

I remember hearing something in a support group that stopped me cold: "What's the last thing you held onto that was just for you?"

Without thinking, my answer was clear earrings.

It was *the* thing that made me feel like myself. Even without makeup. Even without a fresh pedicure. If I had my earrings on, I would feel completely put together. They were my signature. My steadiness. They made me feel like myself. Not just a caregiver, not just a problem-solver, but *me*. Feminine. Grounded. Whole. My small way of saying, I'm still here.

Eventually, I let them go.

Then one day, I didn't. Life got heavy. Too many fires to put out. Too many nights with no sleep. I stopped putting them on. Days turned to weeks. Weeks turned to months. I let go of them without meaning to—and in doing so, I let go of a little piece of myself.

It wasn't about jewelry. It was about the quiet rituals that tether us to who we are beyond caregiving. Those small things matter.

So, if there's something you've let go of—your music, your morning coffee, your favorite jeans—don't feel guilty. Just remember it's okay to come back to yourself. Even in pieces. Even slowly.

A Moment I Will Never Forget – Rest Without Worry

It didn't happen often—two or three times a year—but it meant the world to me. My sister-in-law lived two hours away, but she was the only person we trusted completely with Tre. She didn't just watch him; she understood him. She spoke his language, honored his needs, and loved him in a way that made it safe for us to step away.

Those rare moments of rest were sacred. I wasn't glued to my phone. I wasn't mentally reviewing instructions. I wasn't pacing, anxious, or distracted. I knew he was okay.

For caregivers, real rest only happens when you're not worrying in the background. And because of her, I had that. I had the peace of knowing Tre was not just safe but seen.

It reminded me that rest isn't selfish. It's survival. And when someone steps in with love, it's not just a gift; it's a lifeline.

The Caregiving Mirror – Chapter 10:

What does burnout look like in my life? Are there subtle signs I've been ignoring?

When was the last time I truly felt rested, joyful, or seen? What was different about that moment?

What stories or beliefs do I hold about asking for help or taking a rest? Are they helping or hurting me now?

What's one boundary I've struggled to set—and how might I try again?

Who in my life offers me genuine support or a safe place to rest, even if it's rare?

What's one small act of self-care I can commit to this week, just for me?

If someone I loved were in my shoes, how would I want them to treat themselves?

Your well-being matters too. Support your own well-being with self-care tools at

www.receptivewisdom.com.

Chapter 11
The Self-Care Toolbox

Fundamental Strategies for Real-Life Caregivers

You've probably heard it before: "You have to take care of yourself, too." Easier said than done. Magazines and social media posts often suggest extravagant self-care practices, such as bubble baths and weekend getaways. While these may sound appealing, they're not always feasible for real caregivers. Instead, let's focus on practical, everyday self-care strategies that can be easily incorporated into your routine.

For instance, I couldn't take a weekend off when my daughter was in the hospital. I couldn't go for a walk when Tre was melting down or when Mom had a medication reaction at 2 a.m. So, I had to redefine what self-care looked like—and what it needed to be.

Self-Care Isn't a Luxury—It's Maintenance

It's not selfish.

It's not indulgent.

It's how you *stay in the game.*

You don't owe anyone guilt for taking care of yourself. Because when you go down, the whole system goes down with you. Your rest isn't extra, it's essential.

Their survival often depends on your stability.

Let's get honest about what sustainable self-care looks like when you're caregiving in the real world.

What Realistic Self-Care Looks Like

Let's start with what it's *not*:

A guilt trip

A luxury you "earn" only after everyone else is okay.

Something you put off until the crisis is over.

Instead, it might be:

Ten quiet minutes with your coffee before the day starts.

Listening to music while driving to appointments

Asking for help even if it feels uncomfortable.

Saying no to the negative thoughts that creep into your mind.

The Unintentional Caregiver

Keeping your own doctor's appointment

Letting the dishes wait while you nap.

These aren't grand gestures.

They're life rafts.

What Helped Me (Even When I Had No Time)

These were my fundamental tools. Maybe some will work for you:

Tiny rituals I didn't skip: Lighting the same candle each night. Playing the same playlist during med prep.

A designated safe space: For me, it was the car. Five quiet minutes between errands became a reset.

Texting one trusted person: Not for advice. To say, "It's hard today."

Evening solitude: My recliner. My show. Everyone else is asleep. Just me.

Treating sleep like medicine: Bedtime and naps weren't luxuries. They were doctor's orders.

Doing one thing a week just for me: A podcast. A walk. Writing one paragraph. It reminded me I still existed.

What Didn't Work (and What I Let Go)

Trying to do it all alone

Comparing my story to others

Shaming myself for not doing more

Expecting rest to look "perfect"

I had to stop chasing the fantasy of what self-care "should" look like—and start honoring what actually helped.

If You're Too Tired to Even Try...

That's okay. I've been there many times.

Start tiny.

Drink a glass of water.

Step outside for 60 seconds.

Say one kind thing to yourself—even if you don't fully believe it!

Write down five small things you're grateful for

This isn't about becoming your best self.

It's about preserving yourself, piece by piece, day by day.

Build a Micro-Routine

Even if you don't have an hour, you might have five minutes.

That's where micro-routines come in.

Pick one small action: breathing, journaling, stretching, stepping outside.

Tie it to something you already do brushing teeth, washing dishes, putting your loved one to bed.

Make it non-negotiable—even if it's short.

These tiny rituals anchor your day.

They remind you that you still matter.

Ask Yourself: "What Do I Need Right Now?"

Caregivers are experts at reading everyone else. But when was the last time you asked yourself?

Start checking in with questions like:

Am I hungry, tired, overwhelmed, or lonely?

What would make me feel a little more human right now?

Can something wait until tomorrow?

Your needs won't always come first.

But they should never come last every time.

Boundaries Are a Form of Self-Care

Saying yes to everything will burn you out.

Saying no is sometimes the most loving choice for everyone involved.

Set limits where you can:

On people who constantly take but never support

On responsibilities that aren't truly yours

On your own, perfectionism and guilt

Protecting your energy is not giving up.

It's how you keep going.

Build a Support List

Create a go-to list of people, resources, or activities that lift you up—and keep it visible.

When things feel heavy, use it like a menu:

A friend who listens without judgment

A playlist that helps you breathe

A support group or online forum

A caregiver hotline or therapist

A short walk or moment of stillness

You don't have to do this alone.

And you shouldn't.

A Real Moment of Burnout

I remember one afternoon, sitting in the pharmacy parking lot with meds in the bag beside me, and just... crying. Not because anything new had gone wrong, but because I realized I hadn't eaten all day.

That moment taught me:

Self-care isn't a luxury.

It's fuel. And I'd been running on fumes.

The Self-Care Spectrum

Where You Are, What It Feels Like, Self-Care That Fits

If you are:

Surviving emotionally and physically depleted- Drink water. Breathe. Let something go.

Managing Treading water, heavy but doable. Say no. Step outside. Eat something nourishing.

Rebuilding Slowly Regaining Stability Journal. Nap. Do something joyful.

Thriving Grounded and present Therapy. Dream. Plan something for yourself.

Wherever you are on the spectrum, that place is valid.

Self-care isn't about arriving. It's about responding to your needs with compassion and understanding.

Escape vs. Rest

Zoning out has its place.

But not everything that looks like rest *is* rest.

If it empties you, it's an escape.

If it fills you, it's rest.

Affirmations to Carry with You

I am allowed to rest, even when the work isn't done.

I deserve care without conditions.

I am doing enough, even if it doesn't feel like it.

I am more than what I provide to others.

Reflection Questions

What would I tell a friend in my shoes?

What message is my body trying to send me?

If I could wave a magic wand and receive one kind of support, what would it be?

A Moment I'll Never Forget – Silence and Soil

Some of my most sacred moments came after everyone else had gone to bed. The house was quiet. The TV was on. I wasn't the planner, the advocate, the protector. I was just me.

And then there were the days I stepped outside to dig in the dirt. Gardening wasn't a chore—it was a kind of prayer. Planting something beautiful amid the chaos reminded me:

Life continued to grow, even in the most challenging seasons.

That quiet time—whether watering flowers or sipping coffee in silence—wasn't indulgent. It was survival.

It reminded me that I still mattered.

And in those small rituals, I found my way back to myself.

The Caregiving Mirror – Chapter 11

What's one small act of care I can give myself, without guilt?

What lie have I believed about self-care, and what truth could I replace it with?

Where can I build five minutes of peace this week?

Turn self-care into a practice, not a luxury. Visit www.receptivewisdom.com for checklists, reflection tools, and daily habits you can actually use in real life.

Chapter 12
Life After Caregiving

Rewriting the Story and Honoring the Legacy

Caregiving, by its very nature, demands everything—your time, your emotions, your energy, and sometimes even your identity. But what happens when the calls stop? When the medications are no longer lined up on the counter, or the appointments slow to a halt? What happens when the role shifts… or ends?

No one prepares you for the echo left behind. Whether your caregiving chapter is nearing its close or you're still in it but dreaming of the day when your load is lighter, this space is a realm of freedom and possibility. You are not just a caregiver. You are a person who has carried someone else's world—and now, it's time to explore your own again, with a renewed sense of hope and optimism.

Caregiving changes you, but so does what comes after.

For so long, your life revolved around someone else's needs. Their medication, their appointments, their moods, their safety. And when that season ends, you don't just gain time, you inherit a quiet ache and a whole new set of questions.

Who am I without this role?

What do I do with the habits, the knowledge, the identity I built around caring for someone else?

Some days, you may feel lost, like the version of you that existed before caregiving no longer fits. Other days, you may feel strangely guilty for enjoying a moment of rest or pursuing something just for you.

Let me tell you something with absolute clarity:

You have the right to heal. To rebuild. To dream again.

You are allowed to carry wisdom without carrying the weight.

You are allowed to honor their memory without being consumed by it.

You are allowed to take what caregiving taught you—resilience, tenderness, fierceness, patience—and turn it into something new.

Whether that's advocacy, art, rest, or simply the choice to live a little softer… it all counts.

This next chapter belongs to you. And it doesn't have to be loud, brave, or perfect. It just has to be yours.

"Caregiving" was a chapter of my story, not the whole book. I loved, I served, I gave. And now, I choose to live in a way that honors everything we walked through—together."

Grieving and Gratitude Can Coexist

Some days, the loss will be palpable. It's not just the person you cared for but the daily routine, the sense of purpose, the structure, and the connection.

It's OK to grieve and not miss the chaos. Your feelings are valid and normal. You are not alone on this journey, and it's OK to feel a range of emotions, even those that seem contradictory.

It's OK to feel lighter and not feel guilty.

It's OK to laugh again without apology.

These emotions can coexist without canceling each other out. It's a sign of healing and growth.

Reclaiming Yourself, Intentionally

You may feel lost without the constant demands. That's normal. But this is also your moment to gently begin asking:

Who was I before caregiving?

What parts of me were buried or put on hold?

What passions or strengths surfaced during this time?

Who am I becoming now?

Start small. You don't need to rush into a grand reinvention. Each choice is a tiny act of rediscovery. You are allowed to start over. You are allowed to feel joy again. You are allowed to be more than a caregiver.

Your future is yours to shape, and it holds the promise of joy and satisfaction.

The Person You've Become

You've gained resilience. You've learned how to speak up, how to organize, and how to notice things others miss. You know how to comfort, how to protect yourself, how to manage a dozen things while appearing calm on the outside. These skills are not just remnants of your caregiving days; they are powerful tools that can serve you now and, in the future, empowering you and boosting your confidence.

Those skills? They still belong to you. Let them serve you now—in your work, your relationships, and in how you show up for yourself.

You are more equipped for the next chapter than you realize.

Write a New Chapter for Yourself

This is the moment to ask, gently and without pressure:

What now?

What brings me joy?

What have I put off?

What do I want to feel again?

This doesn't have to mean starting a business or moving across the country—unless that's what you want. Maybe it means reading a book uninterrupted. Dancing in your kitchen. Sitting in silence without rushing to the next thing.

Your future deserves just as much attention as the care you give to others.

Leave a Legacy of Love

You may never get the thank-you you deserve. But caregiving leaves an imprint—not just on the person you loved, but on your family, your community, and your legacy.

Your legacy may be the way your children show up for others. It may be how your story helps another caregiver feel less alone. It may be a quiet strength that lives in the walls of your home.

Your caregiving mattered. It still does.

Giving Yourself Permission

It's OK to move forward without apology.

It's OK to smile without sadness.

It's OK to build a life that's yours again.

You are not abandoning their memory—you are expanding their legacy by continuing to grow and thrive.

Write Your Legacy Letter

Take a moment to reflect on your caregiving journey by writing a letter—

To yourself. To your loved one. Or to another caregiver who might be where you once were.

Include:

What you've learned

What caregiving taught you about love, faith, or strength?

What do you want to carry forward?

It doesn't have to be long or perfect. Let your words honor how far you've come.

The Caregiving Mirror – Chapter 12

Now that my caregiving has ended or shifted, who am I?

What are three things I've always wanted to try—but put off?

What strengths did caregiving uncover in me?

Where in my life do I still need healing?

How can I honor the person I cared for?

How can I share my story to support someone else?

What specific steps can I take to begin my journey of rediscovery?

How do I balance my emotions of grief and joy as I move forward?

What are some practical ways to create a legacy from my caregiving experience?

As you navigate life after caregiving, visit www.receptivewisdom.com for reflection tools, legacy prompts, and gentle ways to honor what came before—while finding hope for what's next.

The Unintentional Caregiver

A Letter to the Next Caregiver

Dear Caregiver,

You probably didn't ask for this.
It could come with a late-night phone call. A diagnosis. A slow decline.

A life that needed holding together when no one else could do it.

Maybe you said, "Of course, I'll help," not realizing that help would become everything. Or perhaps you just looked around one day and realized you were the one holding the medications, making the appointments, interpreting the moods, and keeping someone else alive—emotionally, physically, and spiritually.

If that's where you are, I want you to hear this first: You are not alone.

I wrote this book for you, not as someone who had all the answers, but as someone who had to learn them the hard way. Through hospital visits and school meetings, late-night crying spells, and early-morning victories, I found my way. Not because I was strong, but because I was willing. You might be scared. You might be angry.

It's OK to feel like you're losing yourself in the process of saving someone else. It's OK to feel overwhelmed. These feelings are normal, and they don't diminish the love and care you're giving. That's normal.

You don't have to do it perfectly. You just have to keep showing up.

Remember, you're allowed to take breaks. You're allowed to say no. You're allowed to feel everything and still keep going. But don't forget to take care of yourself. Your well-being is just as important as the care you provide.

The Unintentional Caregiver

You're allowed to say no. You're allowed to feel everything—and still keep going.

And when you don't feel strong? That's OK, too. Strength isn't the absence of struggle—it's continuing through it with love.

You're going to have days where you question everything.

Days when it feels like no one sees what you carry.

But someone does. **I do.**

And so do the many others who've walked this same path, quietly and without applause.

Let this book be your companion, your mirror, and your reminder that what you're doing matters—no matter how messy, how exhausting, or how unappreciated it may be.

And if no one has told you today, **thank you.**

For showing up. For fighting. For loving hard things. You're not just caregiving. You're building something sacred.

Your work is invaluable and deeply appreciated. You are not just caregiving; you are building something sacred. Your dedication and love are shaping a life, a profound and noble task.

With you in spirit and strength,

Joyce Shreve

Author of The Unintentional Caregiver

About the Author

Joyce Shreve didn't set out to become a caregiver, but life had other plans. She stepped into that role first with her mother, whose battle with heart disease taught her how to advocate in hospital rooms and at home. Years later, she would do it all again when her teenage daughter was diagnosed with lupus—and once more when her grandson began his journey with neurodivergence while living with her and her husband.

With no formal training, just love, grit, and a growing pile of medical binders, Joyce became fluent in "doctor-speak," learned to navigate complex systems, and discovered the quiet strength it takes to keep showing up, even when no one is watching.

In *The Unintentional Caregiver*, Joyce opens her story to others walking a similar path. This book is part survival guide, part personal journal, and part love letter to caregivers everywhere. Through it, she offers the support she once wished for—practical tools, honest encouragement, and the reminder that no caregiver is truly alone.

She publishes under the name **Receptive Wisdom**, a phrase that reflects her belief in the kind of clarity that comes only from lived experience, deep listening, and staying soft—even in hard seasons.

When she isn't advocating or sharing her insights with the caregiving community, Joyce can be found enjoying time with her family.

If this book resonated with you, Joyce would love to hear your story. Visit www.receptivewisdom.com to connect.

Acknowledgements

To the doctors, nurses, and medical professionals who gave their time, care, and expertise, thank you. Your knowledge helped save and sustain the people I love most.

To Dr. Mark Mitchiner, Dr. Murray Passo, & Dr. Stacey Cobb. You have been answers to many of my prayers and have blessed our lives more than you will ever know. I'm eternally grateful for your knowledge, bedside manners but most importantly for your care, genuine concern and compassion for your patients. You don't receive the credit and praise you deserve. You are truly amazing human beings, and I am so thankful that our paths crossed. I am a better caregiver because of you. Thank you.

To the speech therapists, especially Mrs. Lindsey, occupational therapists, especially Mrs. Kristen & Mrs. Rachel, RBTs, especially Mrs. Lisa and the BCBAs who worked with Tre: your patience, creativity, and belief in his potential made a difference that can't be measured. You helped him communicate, connect, and grow. You may not remember every visit or every milestone, but we do.

Thank you for being part of our story.

Bonus Materials & Tools

Throughout this book, I've mentioned several tools I've developed and used as caregiver logs, checklists, templates, and organizational aids that made daily caregiving a little more manageable.

Medical Appointment Tracer

Medication and Dosage Log

Emergency Care Binder Cover Sheet

IEP/504 Meeting Preparation Notes

SSI/Medicaid Application Checklist

Daily and Weekly Care Plans

And more

These tools are available on my website. You can also sign up to receive occasional caregiving resources, updates, and support materials that I share exclusively with subscribers. I look forward to connecting with you on your caregiving journey.

Visit www.receptivewisdom.com to access exclusive caregiver tools.

Additional Resources

Here are a few trusted resources that have helped me or come highly recommended by fellow caregivers. Whether you need advocacy tips, emotional support, or guidance navigating complex systems, these organizations and communities offer comfort, clarity, and connection, especially on the days when you feel alone or overwhelmed.

Caregiver Support and Advocacy

Family Caregiver Alliance

www.caregiver.org

Practical tips, fact sheets, and tools to support unpaid caregivers across the U.S.

National Alliance for Caregiving www.caregiving.org

Research, policy initiatives, and advocacy tools for caregivers and professionals.

CaringBridg www.caringbridge.org

A free service that allows families to create private websites to share health updates and coordinate care.

The Mighty – Caregiving Community

www.themighty.com/topic/caregiving

Real-life stories and encouragement from caregivers and people with chronic illnesses.

Medical and Legal Navigation

MedlinePlus www.medlineplus.gov

Plain-language medical information from the U.S. National Library of Medicine.

Disability Rights Education and Defense Fund (DREDF) www.dredf.org

A leading organization advocating for the civil rights of people with disabilities.

Wrights Law www.wrightslaw.com

Guidance and legal information related to special education, IEPs, and parent advocacy.

Neurodivergence and Disability Support

Autism Speaks Toolkit

Practical resources for families supporting individuals with autism, ADHD, and other forms of neurodivergence.

The Arc www.thearc.org

Advocacy and support for individuals with intellectual and developmental disabilities.

Understood.org www.understood.org

Tools and Resources for Parents of Children with Learning and Thinking Differences.

Autistic Self Advocacy Network (ASAN) www.autisticadvocacy.org

Run by and for autistic individuals, ASAN advocates for disability rights and promotes inclusive policy change.

Faith-Based and Holistic Support

Joni and Friends www.joniandfriends.org

Christian ministry offering family retreats, training, and resources for those affected by disability.

Champions Club www.championsclub.org

A church-based special needs ministry model providing spiritual, emotional, and physical support.

Hope Heals www.hopeheals.com

A faith-centered organization sharing stories of resilience, disability, and caregiving through retreats and media.

Community and Local Connections

Local Facebook Caregiver Groups

Search for state or diagnosis-specific caregiver communities in your area for support, tips, and encouragement.

State Medicaid Waiver Programs

Each state offers different waiver programs for home- and community-based services. Search your state's name followed by "Medicaid waiver" for eligibility details.

Parent to Parent USA www.p2pusa.org

Connects parents of children with special needs for one-on-one peer support and mentoring.

The Mighty – Neurodiversity Community

www.themighty.com/topic/neurodiversity

A space to share stories, challenges, and hope with others navigating autism, ADHD, and related conditions.

www.ingramcontent.com/pod-product-compliance
Lightning Source LLC
Chambersburg PA
CBHW060330050426
42449CB00011B/2717